Hardik K. Patel
Rajnikant M. Suthar
Meghana H. Patel

# Handbook of Cosmetic Science and Technology

## The Theory and Practice of Cosmeceuticals

**LAP LAMBERT Academic Publishing**

**Imprint**
Any brand names and product names mentioned in this book are subject to
trademark, brand or patent protection and are trademarks or registered
trademarks of their respective holders. The use of brand names, product
names, common names, trade names, product descriptions etc. even without
a particular marking in this work is in no way to be construed to mean that
such names may be regarded as unrestricted in respect of trademark and
brand protection legislation and could thus be used by anyone.

Cover image: www.ingimage.com

Publisher:
LAP LAMBERT Academic Publishing
is a trademark of
International Book Market Service Ltd., member of OmniScriptum Publishing
Group
17 Meldrum Street, Beau Bassin 71504, Mauritius

Printed at: see last page
**ISBN: 978-3-659-66550-9**

Copyright © Hardik K. Patel, Rajnikant M. Suthar, Meghana H. Patel
Copyright © 2015 International Book Market Service Ltd., member of
OmniScriptum Publishing Group
All rights reserved. Beau Bassin 2015

## PREFACE

Cosmetic composition and formulation are becoming increasingly complex, and cosmetic ingredients more sophisticated and functional, while laws and regulations impose more constraints on the cosmetic scientist and manufacturer. The *Handbook of Cosmetic Science and Technology* reviews in a single volume the multiple facets of the cosmetic field and provides the reader with an easy-to-access information source.

This handbook covers topics as varied as the physiology of the potential targets of cosmetics, safety, legal and regulatory considerations throughout the world, cosmetic ingredients, vehicles and finished products, and new delivery systems, as well as microbiology and safety and efficacy testing.

To achieve our goal, we, the authors, requested the contributions of expert scientists from academic dermatology and dermato-cosmetics, the cosmetics industry, ingredients and raw materials producers, and regulatory agencies. We thank the editors for their high dedication, which permitted us to make this handbook a review of the state of the art in cosmetology in the new millennium.

Finally, we encourage our readership to send us their comments and suggestions on what should be modified or considered in future editions.

*HARDIK K. PATEL*
*RAJNIKANT M. SUTHAR*
*MEGHANA H. PATEL*

## ACKNOWLEDGEMENT

First, I would like to express my salutation to **GOD** for giving me the strength, confidence and moral boost to successful completion of this book.

"You want to do the right thing and you want to do it for the right reasons but if you don't have the right guidance you can never hit the right target." It is great pleasure and profound sense of reverence that I express my gratitude and thank to my Head of Department **Dr. (Mrs) J. R. Parikh** for his eruptive guidance, suggestion and encouragement during this and other project works. This work would have been impossible without her constant support and total understanding.

I also pass a special vote of thanks to **Dr. A. K. Saluja,** Principal of college for providing me the infrastructure and research facilities at the college for conducting my study. I owe a special word of thanks to my all other colleague teachers for extending their help during the course of investigation.

I am thankful to **my parents** who led me from darkness to light, ignorance to enlighten and confusion to clarity throughout my life. I shall forever be grateful to my dearest brothers and sister **Nikunj, Jitu, Viral** and **Anjali** for their sweet deposition, motivation to work and their admirable help during entire course of my project work.

"Your sorrows get divided and your happiness get multiplied with your friends." A friend is a person who understands your filling, emotion and helps you to be what you to be. I am thankful to all my friends who helped me in hardship through the sweet fragrance of friendship without which I could not have won all the battles.

I would also like to thank **Mr. Rupesh Patel** computer laboratory assistant, **Mrs. Parul Patel** and library staff to support me a lot.

"May the candle be lightened forever, the joy is not of light alone, but of presence of those, who played the role behind the curtain."

*HARDIK K. PATEL*
*M. Pharm, MBA*

# CONTENTS

- Preface (i)
- Acknowledgement (ii)
- (1) Introduction: Cosmetic 01 – 02
- (2) Cosmetics for skin 03 – 44
  - (A) Powder preparations
    - a) Face powder
    - b) Compacts
      - i) Cake make-up powders
      - ii) Liquid and cream powders
      - iii) Cosmetic stocking
    - c) Toilet powders
      - i) Talcum powder
      - ii) Dusting powder
      - iii) After shave powder
      - iv) Baby powder
  - (B) Cream preparations
    - a) Cold creams
    - b) Cleansing creams
    - c) All purpose creams
    - d) Lubricating or emollient creams
    - e) Skin protective and hand creams
    - f) Vanishing creams
    - g) Foundation creams
    - h) Liquid creams
    - i) Miscellaneous creams
      - i) Acid creams
      - ii) Bleaching creams
      - iii) Astringent creams

- (C) Lotion preparations
  - a) Hand lotions
  - b) Skin toning lotions
  - c) Astringent lotions
  - d) Bleaching and freckle lotions
  - e) After shave lotions
- (D) Miscellaneous preparations
  - a) Deodorants
  - b) Bathing preparations
  - c) Make up preparations
    - i) Rouges
    - ii) Mascara
    - iii) Eye shadows
    - iv) Eyebrow pencils
    - v) Lipsticks

(3) Cosmetics for hair and shaving media     45 – 56
  - a) Shampoos
  - b) Scalp and dandruff tonics
  - c) Brilliantines and hair dressings
  - d) Hair washing preparations
  - e) Depilatories
  - f) Pre-shaving lotions
  - g) Shaving media

(4) Cosmetics for nails     57 – 58

(5) Dentifrices     59 – 62

- Bibliography     63

# 1. INTRODUCTION: COSMETIC

**Introduction: Cosmetic**

Now a days, 'Cosmetic' is not an uncommon thing for human beings. It has become more or less a necessary requirement in daily life for any part of the body, may be for skin, hair or nails. People have been using cosmetics since ancient times for beautifying, promoting attractiveness, altering the appearance and for the care of body, eyes, teeth, hair, face, etc. Thus, cosmetics are mainly used for two purposes, i.e. care of body parts and enhancing personal appeal of human beings.

The consumption of cosmetics becomes immensely large since toilet soaps and dental preparations (tooth powder and paste) have been included in cosmetics. Recently, more and more people are becoming regular user of the cosmetic preparations. Thus, for legal control, its manufacturing has been governed under the Drugs and Cosmetics Act, 1940 and defined as follows:

"Any article intended to be rubbed, poured, sprinkled or sprayed on or introduced into or otherwise applied to the human body or over part thereof for cleaning, beautifying, promoting attractiveness or altering the appearance".

**Classification of Cosmetics:**

Cosmetics are classified under two main groups:

**Group – I:** According to the part of organ of the body on which they are to be used.

**Group – II:** According to their physical nature.

Group – I is further subdivided as follows:

a) For skin: e.g. Powders, creams, lotions, deodorants, bath and cleansing preparation, Make-up, suntan preparations etc.
b) For hair: e.g. Shampoos, tonics, hair dressings and brillantines, hair waving, beard softner, shaving media, depilatories, etc.
c) For nails: e.g. Nail poish and its removers, manicure preparations etc.
d) For teeth and mouth: e.g. Dentifrices, mouth washes etc.

# Introduction: Cosmetic

Group – II is further divided as follows:

a) Aerosols: e.g. Perfumes, hair set, hair sprays etc.
b) Cakes: e.g. Rouge, Compact shaving cake, toilet soap etc.
c) Emulsions: e.g. Cold cream, vanishing cream, cleansing creams etc.
d) Jellies: e.g. Hand jelly, wave set jelly, brilliantine jelly etc.
e) Mucilages: e.g. Wave set, hand lotion etc.
f) Oils: e.g. Brilliantine, hair oils etc.
g) Pastes: e.g. Tooth paste, deodorants paste etc.
h) Powders: e.g. Face powder, tooth powder, talcum powder etc.
i) Solutions: e.g. Shampoos, after shave lotion, astringent lotion etc.
j) Sticks: e.g. Lipsticks, deodorant sticks etc.
k) Suspensions: e.g. Liquid powder, lotions etc.

## 2. COSMETICS FOR SKIN

**Cosmetics for Skin:**

Cosmetics for skin are further classified as follows:

- a) Powder preparations
- b) Cream preparations
- c) Lotions preparations
- d) Miscellaneous preparations

a) **Powder preparations:**
   1) Face powder
   2) Compacts
      i) Cake make-up powders
      ii) Liquid and cream powders
      iii) Cosmetic stocking
   3) Toilet powders
      i) Talcum powders
      ii) Dusting powders
      iii) After shave powders
      iv) Baby powders

b) **Cream preparations:**
   1) Cold creams
   2) Cleansing creams
   3) All purpose creams
   4) Lubricating or emollient creams
   5) Skin protective and hand creams
   6) Vanishing creams
   7) Foundation creams
   8) Liquid creams
   9) Miscellaneous creams
      i) Acid creams
      ii) Bleaching creams
      iii) Astringent creams

# Cosmetics for Skin

c) **Lotions preparations:**
   1) Hand lotions
   2) Skin toning lotions
   3) Skin freshners
   4) Astringent lotions
   5) Bleaching and freckle lotions
   6) After shave lotions

d) **Miscellaneous preparations:**
   1) Deodorants
   2) Bathing preparations
   3) Make-up preparations
      i) Rouges
      ii) Mascara
      iii) Eye shadows
      iv) Eyebrow pencils
      v) Lipsticks

**Face Powder:**

Now a days, face powder becomes very much popular in women section to improve the personal attractiveness. Men are also not uncommon to use the face powder for covering up the need of shave temporarily or applies after shave to improve their own personality.

Since women are the maximum user of face powder, their requirements be given careful consideration. Two important needs for them are, proper colour and proper smell. These two characteristics are the prime factors in improving the sell of face powder among women. Additionally, face powder must possess following characteristics:

- Very fine particle size and should not have any gritty particles.
- Easily and evenly distributed on the skin.
- No irritability and toxicity to the skin.
- Chemically and physically stable.
- Easily adhered to the skin.
- Good absorbing property.
- Able to remove shine from the oily face.

# Cosmetics for Skin

- Able to cover minor imperfections of the face.
- Ability to be retained on the face for longer period.

Thus, to provide all these characteristics following ingredients are required in the manufacturing of face powder:

1) Covering powders to conceal shine and minor skin imperfections, ingredients like Titanium dioxide, Zinc oxide, Zinc sulphide, Lithopone, Kaolin (Colloidal), Calcium sulphate, Magnesium oxide, Starch etc. are used for this purpose.
2) Some ingredients which provide ease and smooth application to the skin, e.g. Talc, Starch, Metallic soaps.
3) It is necessary to make the powder sufficiently adhesive so that it will remain on the skin for a quite reasonable time. This requirement of the powder is fulfilled by adding ingredients like Calcium, Magnesium and Zinc stearate, Starch and Colloidal clays (Purified Kaolin).
4) Face powder must possess some ingredients which acts as a binder for the colour and perfumes. Binder facilitates the uniform distribution of colour and perfume throughout the bulk of the powder.

The principal materials which are commonly incorporated in the formulation of powder are Zinc oxide, Titanium dioxide, Talc, Kaolin, the Stearates, Starch and Chalk.

Few formulae are given to prepare face powder using Zinc oxide, Purified Kaolin, Titanium dioxide and combination of Zinc oxide and Titanium dioxide as a covering agents.

| Formula – I: Light Face Powder | |
|---|---|
| Zinc oxide | : 18 gm |
| Talc | : 67.52 gm |
| Zinc stearate | : 6 gm |
| Precipitated chalk | : 6 gm |
| Perfume | : 1 gm |
| Ochre | : 1.44 gm |
| Brilliant pink lake | : 0.04 gm |

**Formula – II: Medium Face Powder**

| | |
|---|---|
| Titanium dioxide | : 4 gm |
| Purified kaolin | : 20 gm |
| Talc | : 64.52 gm |
| Magnesium stearate | : 3 gm |
| Magnesium carbonate | : 6 gm |
| Perfume | : 1 ml |
| Ochre | : 1.44 gm |
| Brilliant pink lake | : 0.04 gm |

**Formula – III: Medium Face Powder**

| | |
|---|---|
| Titanium dioxide | : 5.21 gm |
| Talc | : 81.31 gm |
| Zinc stearate | : 5 gm |
| Precipitated chalk | : 6 gm |
| Perfume | : 1 ml |
| Ochre | : 1.44 gm |
| Brilliant pink lake | : 0.04 gm |

**Formula – IV: Heavy Face Powder**

| | |
|---|---|
| Titanium dioxide | : 3 gm |
| Zinc oxide | : 20 gm |
| Talc | : 64.52 gm |
| Zinc stearate | : 6 gm |
| Precipitated chalk | : 7 gm |
| Perfume | : 7 ml |
| Ochre | : 1.44 gm |
| Brilliant pink lake | : 0.04 gm |

The stepwise method of preparation for preparing all the above powders is given below:

- Mix perfume with a part of magnesium carbonate or the chalk in a suitable vessel.
- Rub the mixture through a hand sieve with a stiff bristle till the perfume is uniformly distributed.
- Mix the colour in the same way with the rest of the magnesium carbonate or chalk.
- Continue mixing the colour mixture until a portion rubbed out on a white paper shows on colour flecks. Keep a sample for matching successive bathces.
- Weigh out and put the rest of the raw materials into a mixer, add the perfume and colour base and mix until uniform.
- Take the sample and rub it out on white paper, it should not show any colour flecks on the paper.
- Match the sample with the previous batch sample. If it matches, then stop mixing otherwise, continue till it is completely matched without any line of demarcation.
- Finally sift the powder through sieve no. 160 and fill in a proper container.

One more method is common to prepare face powders in which the whole method is divided into two operations. First the preparation of white powder base, which is perfumed and stored in light bins to age and mellow the perfume. During this time perfume will permeate through each particle of the base material. Second operation is to prepare colour base and stored. At the time of manufacturing face powder, required amount of white powder base and colour base are weighed and mix until uniform. This particular method speeds up the manufacturing of face powder with successive uniform batches.

**Compacts:**

Compacts include; compact powder, cake make-up powders, cream and liquid powders. They are very close in composition to face powders.

Cosmetics stocking are also included in this category since they are close to the liquid powders.

A compact powder is a face powder which has been compacted into a cake, properly packed in a suitable container along with a powder puff for its application on face. The advantage of compact powder is that large bulk of the powder is reduced by compression into cake form. The characteristics of compact powder are more or less same as in case of face powder, i.e. all requirements like slip, adhesion, covering powder, colour and odour. Since it is a compact cake which must neither be too hard nor too soft. The powder must come off easily on the puff and the cake must not get hard and shiny.

Basic materials required to manufacture compact powder are also same as those of face powder, i.e. talc, kaolin, colloidal clay, bentonite, zinc oxide, titanium dioxide, precipitated chalk, magnesium carbonate and stearate of zinc, aluminium and magnesium. Pigments, lakes and colours are also same as in face powder.

To avoid the cracking or breaking of cakes, talc is restricted upto 50%. The binding solution is also required to bind the powder mixture into damp mass before either granulation or compaction as the case may be. Binding solution is a mucilage made from materials like gelatin, gum tragacanth, gum acacia, gum karay, methyl cellulose, quince seed, rosin, irish moss etc. Sometimes lanolin dissolved in ether is used for this purpose.

There are mainly three methods of compression:

1) Wet compression
2) Dry compression
3) Wet casting process

The first two methods are same as in the manufacturing of tablet, so here we do not discuss them in detail. The wet casting process consists of making a wet, heavy paste of the powder mixture. The paste is poured or passed by rolling into lubricated nickel moulds, in which cakes are dried completely. The important point which must be taken care of is painting of surface of cakes with dextrin or gum Arabic adhesive and pressing of either glass, porcelain or metal plate over glued surface of the cakes, just before putting them in dryer. When cakes are dried, they are sticked to the plates.

# Cosmetics for Skin

A typical formula for binding solution is given below:

| | |
|---|---|
| Gum tragacanth mucilage (2%) | : 20 % |
| Quince seed mucilage (2%) | : 10 % |
| Gelatin mucilage (3%) | : 10 % |
| Rosin tincture | : 1 % |
| Purified water | : 58.8 % |
| Methyl para hydroxy benzoate | : 0.2 % |

A typical compact powder can be prepared by the following formula:

| | |
|---|---|
| Talc (300 mesh) | : 30 gm |
| Zinc oxide | : 25 gm |
| Zinc stearate | : 11 gm |
| Rice sarch | : 10 gm |
| Magnesium carbonate | : 3 gm |
| Colloidal clay | : 10 gm |
| Colour pigments | : 10.5 gm |
| Perfume | : 0.5 ml |

Mix all the ingredients of the formula and run through a pulverizer, or a ball mill. Moisten the powder with a sufficient quantity of the binding solution to make damp mass and then pass it through a proper sieve to form granules. Granules are dried completely in an oven and then dried granules are again compressed to form a cake.

Recently cake make-up which are designated as pan cake make-up, becoming very popular. It has advantages to produce flat, smooth, enduring finish to the skin that can not be acquired by any other cosmetic. At the same time it conceals minor skin imperfections.

In manufacture and formulation of cake make-up, care must be taken to keep formula and processing standardised. Unless the processes are kept uniform an inferior product will result. Addition of colours must be carefully done so that uniformity is maintained from batch to batch.

Materials used for cake make up are just like those as in face powders, e.g. talc, chalk, kaolin, colloidal clay, titanium dioxide and zinc oxide. These materials are in addition to light or heavy mineral oils, vegetable oils, pigments, perfumes, water, humectants like glycerol and glycols, binding and emulsifying agents.

It should have following characteristics:

- It should come off easily with a moistened applicator or sponge, as an emulsion or by some other medium.
- It should lay on the skin uniformly.
- The film formed on the skin should not come off through rapid drying. It should stay on the skin during the whole day.
- It should repel the moisture caused by perspiration.
- It should be readily removed by washing with soap and water.

Mineral earths play an important role in order to possess the desirable properties. Titanium dioxide and zinc oxide impart covering and masking properties to the cake, kaolin and colloidal clay help as binders in compressing. Chalk regulates the ease of brushing off or blending with the skin. Talc is more or less a stable filler. A formulator must use a combination of these ingredients for the desired effect.

The oils are added to produce the desired amount of oiliness. Mineral oils are stable but vegetable oils should be stabilized with an antioxidant. Numerous emulsifying agents are available in incorporate in the formulation. The amount of emulsifying agents must not be more than required otherwise it may over dry the skin by degreasing it.

The method of preparation is to add water/oil emulsion and humectant in the mixture of powders. This will form a paste which is passed through a roll mixer to obtain a homogenity. This paste is then granulated and pressed into cakes.

Liquid and cream powders, also called 'night whites' are used for evening wear to offset the glare of electric light. These preparations are applied to face, neck and arms. Because of their high opacity they serves to cover the colour of skin exposed in evening.

# Cosmetics for Skin

| Formula – I: Liquid Powder | |
|---|---|
| Colloidal clay | : 18 gm |
| Titanium dioxide | : 2 gm |
| Glycerine | : 8 ml |
| Water | : 71.5 ml |
| Perfume | : 0.5 ml |

| Formula – II: Liquid Powder | |
|---|---|
| Talc | : 10 gm |
| Colloidal clay | : 5 gm |
| Titanium dioxide | : 5 gm |
| Glycerine | : 10 ml |
| Rose water | : 64 ml |
| Alcohol | : 5.5 ml |
| Perfume | : 0.5 ml |

Method of preparation of liquid powder is simple. Mix all the powder materials in a powder mixer. The liquid ingredients are blended in suitable vessel which is preferably equipped with a mechanical agitator. The powders are added to the blended liquids slowly with the agitator. After all the powders have been added the mass is stirred for about half an hour. The finished liquid powder is then filled in a suitable container. Continuous agitation is required during filling operation to restrict the settling of solids.

| Formula – III: Cream Powder | |
|---|---|
| Glyceryl Monostearate | : 10 ml |
| Glycerin | : 2 ml |
| Heavy mineral oil | : 5 ml |
| Spermaceti | : 5 ml |
| Stearic acid | : 2 gm |
| Caustic potash | : 0.1 ml |
| Water | : 48.5 ml |
| Perfume | : 0.4 ml |

# Cosmetics for Skin

| Titanium dioxide | : 7 gm |
| Talc | : 20 gm |

Dissolve the caustic potash in water and add all other ingredients except perfume. Include colour (if present). Heat the mixture to boil with constant stirring. Continue stirring till all the waxy materials melt and form a homogeneous mass. Heating is stopped and stirring is continued till the mass cooled, then add perfume. Pass the final mass through roller mill to obtain a uniform product.

One more type of preparation included in this class is cosmetic stockings which are hardly face powders but their physical form is so close to the liquid face powder and hence feel necessity to discuss here. Cosmetic stocking are the leg make-up which provide bare legs the artificial texture like appearance of women's hose.

The requirements for cosmetic stockings are the colours simulating the popular shades of women's hose; alcohol for rapid drying; glycerin, sorbitol, propylene glycol for providing emollient effect on the skin and a little wetting agent for even deposition of the colour. Colloidal clay e.g. bentonite is added to keep the pigments in suspended form for a longer time. Talc is used to provide the luster to the mixture, permitting better simulation of silk texture. A little amount of gum is needed to make the powder adhere firmly to the skin surface.

| Formula – IV: Liquid Cosmetic Stocking | |
|---|---|
| Precipitated chalk | : 10 gm |
| Talc | : 5 gm |
| Titanium dioxide | : 3 gm |
| Bentonite | : 2 gm |
| Alcohol | : 8 ml |
| Glycerine | : 3 ml |
| Wetting agent | : 0.5 ml |
| Methyl cellulose | : 0.5 gm |
| Water | : 68 ml |
| Dye and pigment | : q.s. |

# Cosmetics for Skin

Mix all the powder ingredients except dye in a powder mixer. Mix all liquid ingredients in a separate vessel in which it is feasible to fit a mechanical stirrer. Dissolve the dye in a liquid mixture and add powder mixture in parts with the help of stirrer. When all the powder mixture has been added then continues stirring for at least half an hour for getting homogeneous product.

**Toilet Powders:**

Toilet powders are more extravagantly used over large surfaces of the body than face powders. They comprise of talcum powder, dusting powder, after shave powder and baby powder.

The most important is the talcum powder. Talc is the main component of talcum powder. It varies from 60 to 90 percent. The other ingredients used are zinc stearate, zinc oxide, light magnesium carbonate, magnesium stearate, light calcium carbonate, precipitated chalk, boric acid etc.

Zinc stearate provides soothing and mild antiseptic properties. Zinc oxide acts as a mild astringent and relieves the prickling and irritation. Magnesium stearate provides good slip to the powder. Light calcium or magnesium carbonate increases fluffiness of the talcum powder.

The function of talcum powder is to absorb perspiration, absorb moisture after bath and allay irritation of the skin due to chafing.

The talc must be of high quality and should possess following characteristics:

1) It must be white.
2) It must possess adequate slip properties to facilitate spreading over skin.
3) It should be lustrous and free from grittiness.
4) It should be sterilized.

# Cosmetics for Skin

| Formula – I: Talcum Powder | |
|---|---|
| Talc | : 74 gm |
| Precipitated chalk | : 18 gm |
| Zinc stearate | : 2 gm |
| Boric acid | : 5 gm |
| Perfume | : 1 ml |

| Formula – II: Talcum Powder | |
|---|---|
| Talc | : 80 gm |
| Magnesium carbonate | : 12 gm |
| Boric acid | : 5 gm |
| Magnesium stearate | : 2 gm |
| Perfume | : 1 ml |

Mix the perfume with part of the magnesium carbonate or the chalk powder and colour (if present) in the remaining part of these powders. If colour is not present in the formula, take whole of the amount for distributing perfume. Pass the mixture through sieve until the perfume and colour are uniformly distributed.

Weigh out the rest of the raw materials into a mixer, add the perfume and colour base, mix until uniform.

Dusting powder, after shave powder and baby powder are very closely related to the talcum powder. All these have more or less the same composition as the talcum powder. Dusting powder is usually applied with a puff to body of the person. After shave powder consists of talc to which has been added the colour and some other mineral ingredients to spread smoothly, cling to the face with less sheen and more nearly the colour of men's flesh. Baby powder is usually less perfumed than other toilet powder and without colour. An important ingredients which must be added not only to baby powder but to all toilet powders is boric acid because of its soothing and slightly antiseptic properties.

# Cosmetics for Skin

| Formula – III: After Shave Powder | |
|---|---|
| Talc | : 75 gm |
| Titanium dioxide | : 4 gm |
| Zinc stearate | : 4 gm |
| Precipitated chalk | : 15.5 gm |
| Golden ochre | : 0.5 gm |
| Perfume | : 1 ml |

| Formula – IV: Baby Powder | |
|---|---|
| Talc | : 70.75 gm |
| Magnesium carbonate | : 8 gm |
| Colloidal clay | : 8 gm |
| Magnesium stearate | : 4 gm |
| Boric acid | : 10 gm |
| Titanium dioxide | : 3 gm |
| Perfume | : 0.25 ml |

Follow the method of preparation as in case of talcum powder.

**Cream Preparations:**

Cosmetic creams are becoming more and more popular because of their various advantages. Since they are emulsions and can be available in either o/w or w/o form which may provide the opportunity to choose the cream for oily or for dry skin respectively. They are less greasy than the oleaginous preparations which render them products of first choice of users. They cover variety of functions which are required for skin care as well as for make up purposes. For streamline discussion they are classified and discussed as follows:

a) **Cold Creams:**

The 'Cold cream' is named after its function which provide cooling effect on application due to the evaporation of water separated by breaking of w/o emulsion. It has been found as a most popular preparation since long back and still its popularity is not being diminished instead flourished.

# Cosmetics for Skin

The most popular cold cream (water – in – oil emulsion) is prepared by using bees wax water and alkali, usually borax, the bees wax possesses few free fatty acids which reacts with borax and form the esters of fatty acids, functioning as an emulsifying agent to emulsify water with wax or oil. So, for any cream, basically three things are required i.e. aqueous phase, oily phase and an emulsifying agent. The volume of phase will decide the type of emulsion or cream. The phase which is in large amount will always form the continuous phase. An emulsifying agent can be added as one of the ingredients or can be prepared in situ. In cold cream, the internal phase of an emulsion is aqueous, while external phase is oily.

Cold creams are used as emollient creams and are useful for dry skin. They are quite popular in winter season.

**Formula – I: Cold Cream**

| | |
|---|---|
| Spermaceti | : 4 gm |
| White bees wax | : 15 gm |
| White mineral oil (65 – 75) | : 56 ml |
| Borax | : 0.8 gm |
| Distilled water | : 23.7 ml |
| Perfume | : 0.5 ml |

**Formula – II: Cold Cream**

| | |
|---|---|
| White bees wax | : 20 gm |
| White mineral oil (65 – 75) | : 50 gm |
| Distilled water | : 28.8 ml |
| Borax | : 0.7 gm |
| Perfume | : 0.5 ml |

Dissolve the borax in hot water. Separately melt all the waxy materials and oils are added to it. Heat the molten mass at about 70°C. Pour in the borax solution at the same temperature with constant stirring until cold. When the temperature is dropped to about 45°C - 50°C, add the perfume.

Triethanolamine can be employed as an alkali in place of borax. A little variation is to be made in the method of preparation,

Melt waxes, fats and oils together, bring the temperature to about 80°C. Then take water, glycerine and triethanolamine in another beaker and bring the solution almost to the boiling point. Add the melted fat to triethanolamine solution. Stir continuously until cold. Perfume is added when the temperature is lowered to 45°C - 50°C.

Cold creams containing glyceryl monostearate are easy to manufacture. Since it is self emulsifying agent, all the ingredients in the formula are put into a vessel and heated to the boiling point with constant stirring. When all the material get melting, stop heating further but stirring is continued until cold. When the temperature is lowered to about 45 – 50°C, add perfume.

Cold creams made with borax are superior to those without it, since the emulsion is whiter, smoother and more stable.

**b) Cleansing Creams:**

Cleansing cream is water-in-oil emulsion used to clean the dirt on the skin. The dirt on the skin consists of residues of skin secretions as well as deposits from the surroundings. The dirt can be washed off by the soap, but it is not advisable since it might have drying effect on the skin surface due to excess alkali present in the soap. Thus in order to remove the dirt instead of emulsification process due to residual oils on the skin surface soap and water, solvent action of mineral oil is exploited to remove the skin dirt. A cleansing cream must possess following characteristics:

i) It should liquefy at body temperature.
ii) It should have low viscosity so as to spread easily but high enough to retain dirt particles.
iii) It should penetrate the epidermis via natural openings and permit flushing the pores.
iv) It should leave the skin smooth, relaxed, refreshed, nongreasy and clean.

Mineral oil is an essential ingredients of all the cleansing creams.

# Cosmetics for Skin

| Formula – I: Liquefying Cleansing Cream ||
|---|---|
| Beeswax | : 4 gm |
| Paraffin | : 10 gm |
| White petrolatum | : 10.8 gm |
| Mineral oil | : 55.0 ml |
| Purified water | : 18 ml |
| Borax | : 1.2 gm |
| Glycerin | : 1 ml |

| Formula – II: Cleansing Cream ||
|---|---|
| Bees wax | : 8 gm |
| Paraffin | : 5 ml |
| Petrolatum | : 7.4 gm |
| Mineral oil | : 44.8 ml |
| Borax | : 0.3 gm |
| Purified Water | : 34.5 ml |

Follow the methods for the above two preparations as in cold cream.

c) **All Purpose Creams:**

All purpose cream is a cream which combines the properties of specialized creams. As such any cold cream or cleansing cream with little additional or extended uses is termed as all purpose cream. It can be used as emollient, cleansing and foundation creams.

| Formula – I: All Purpose Cream ||
|---|---|
| Water | : 35 ml |
| Borax | : 1 gm |
| Beeswax | : 8 gm |
| Iso beeswax | : 6 gm |
| Ceresin | : 3 gm |
| Absorption base | : 3 gm |
| Mineral oil (S.G.O. 910) | : 44 ml |
| Perfume | : …q.s… |

Dissolve borax in water. Melt all waxes, absorption base and mineral oil together in a separate beaker. Heat both the phases, i.e. aqueous and oily, in a water bath to nearly 70°C and then aqueous phase is added to oily phase with constant stirring. Stirring is continued. When the temperature cools down to nearly 40 - 45°C, perfume is added to the cream with again constant stirring.

### d) Lubricating or Emollient Creams:

Lubricating creams are widely popular for dry skin. The skin is not only dried out by exposure to the sun, wind and salt air in summer but also becomes dry and roughened in the winter by the low humidity in the environment. Thus, the lubricating creams have their use to supply oils to dried skins which are deficient in oil.

Lanolin is found much useful in adding into the formulation of lubricating creams since it is obtained from the animal source and contains some of the same constituents that are secreted by the sebaceous glands of the human skin.

A lubricating cream should possess the following properties:

i) It should spread easily.
ii) It should have fine texture.
iii) It should have good skin absorption.
iv) It should not be sticky in nature.
v) It should be smooth in nature with less oiliness.

The commonly used materials for preparing lubricating cream are lanolin, cetyl alcohol, beeswax, petrolatum, stearic acid, animal or vegetable oils and fats, spermaceti, fatty alcohols, glyceryl monostearate and other fatty acid esters, sorbitol esters and absorption bases. Sometimes, pure cholesterin and vegetable lecithin are also added.

It is very important to find out the proper amount of lanolin which is quite sticky itself otherwise, it may turn the cream sticky which is not easily and smoothly applied over the skin. The consistency of the cream can be adjusted by changing the amount of oil, wax and water in the formula. Whenever vegetable or animal substances are used, a preservatives and antioxidant must be added.

# Cosmetics for Skin

| Formula – I: Lubricating Cream with Cholesterin ||
|---|---|
| Cocoa butter (Odourless) | : 8 gm |
| Beeswax (White) | : 20 gm |
| Cetyl alcohol | : 2 gm |
| Mineral oil, white | : 44.3 ml |
| Cholesterin (Pure) | : 2.5 gm |
| Borax | : 1 gm |
| Purified water | : 21 ml |
| Methyl paraben | : 0.2 gm |
| Perfume | : ...q.s... |

First melt fats and waxes in a beaker, add mineral oil and cholesterin, stir. In another beaker, dissolve borax and methyl paraben in water. Heat both the phases on a water bath. When the temperature of both the phases becomes nearly same (about 70°C), add aqueous phase into oily phase gently with constant stirring. Continue stirring until the temperature drops to 45 - 50°C and then add the perfume. Mix thoroughly until it is uniformly mixed.

| Formula – II: Cold Cream base Lubricating Cream ||
|---|---|
| White petrolatum | : 35 gm |
| Beeswax (White) | : 11 gm |
| Spermaceti | : 4 gm |
| Lanolin | : 4 gm |
| White mineral oil | : 34 ml |
| Borax | : 0.5 gm |
| Methyl paraben | : 0.1 gm |
| Perfume | : ...q.s... |

First, melt the fats and wax and then add oil, bring the temperature of the mixture to nearly 70°C. Dissolve the borax in water in a separate beaker and bring its temperature to the same as of oily phase. Add the borax solution to the oily phase with constant stirring. Continue mixing until the temperature drops to 45 - 50°C, then add the perfume. Dissolve the methyl paraben in a little alcohol and mix into the batch.

### e) Skin protective and Hand Creams:

Skin protective creams are developed for those persons who are working in such industries where their skin come across many hazardous chemicals and environmental conditions which may promote different skin diseases. These creams protect the skin if applied before entering to such environment and handling sort of chemicals.

Many industrial chemicals are known capable of producing occupational dermatitis in the personnels working there. They may be acids, alkalis, hypertonic solutions, soaps, gases, vapours, fat solvents, cement, plaster, dye, metallic oxide and hot water. These substances may show their harmful effect due to:

- Dissolving the horney layer.
- Dissolving the protective natural grease on the skin.
- Protein precipitation.
- Desiccation.
- Dissociation or hydrolysis in water to form irritating compounds.
- Oxidation.
- Reduction.

These harmful effects depend on various factors; the character of the substance, the concentration and degree of exposure to the irritant.

Protective substances can be classified into four groups. The first group includes fats and oils such as petrolatum jelly, lanolin, wax, etc. These are quite popular but have disadvantages like staining of skin, require strong detergents for their removal, which may in turn induce dermatitis.

The second group consists of starch, tragacanth, agar, glycerine and honey. These substances do not exert protective action but forms a barrier film. They do not adhere for long enough since they are readily soluble in water and are highly absorptive.

The third group consists of emulsions which are formed by the combination of ingredients of first and second groups. Emulsions are the most suitable form of the cream which can be easily applied on skin leaving a fatty barrier on it. They also requires soaps to remove them.

# Cosmetics for Skin

The fourth group consists of substances like soap bases, like the alkaline salts or stearate, oleates and palmitates. The chief disadvantage of these substances is the chances of skin irritation due to presence of free alkalis.

An ideal protective cream must have the following characteristics:

i) It must be spread easily.
ii) It must remain stable in the presence of most other chemical agents.
iii) It must provide an oil film of low surface tension.
iv) It must not be hygroscopic.
v) It must be absorbed into the skin upto some extent.
vi) It must be easy to remove without the use of detergents, soaps or scrubbing-brushes.

| Formula: Protective Cream | |
|---|---|
| Glyceryl monostearate | : 8 gm |
| Magnesium stearate | : 14 gm |
| Beeswax | : 3 gm |
| Petrolatum | : 9 gm |
| Mineral oil | : 6 ml |
| Water | : 60 ml |

Take all the ingredients in a beaker and heat on a water bath upto 70°C. Stir until cold.

Hand creams are modified vanishing creams. Physically, hand creams are little harder but must be readily spread and must not show any rolling. A large amount of glycerine is added in these types of creams to avoid any rolling tendencies. Hand creams should be:

i) Greaseless and easily rubbed without rolling.
ii) Non sticky.
iii) Able to alleviate chap of the skin.

Materials used in the hand creams to soften and soothe the skin include cetyl alcohol, cocoa butter, tincture of benzoin, lecithin, mucilage of quince seed or karaya etc. If gums are added to the creams, it is necessary to add preservatives like methyl or butyl esters of parahydroxy-benzoic acid.

# Cosmetics for Skin

| Formula: Hand Cream | |
|---|---|
| Cetyl alcohol | : 1.5 gm |
| Stearic acid | : 15.5 gm |
| Cocoa butter | : 3 gm |
| Triethanolamine | : 1.75 gm |
| Glycerine | : 17.5 ml |
| Alcohol | : 6 ml |
| Water | : 52.6 ml |
| Quince seed | : 1.5 gm |
| Perfume | : ...q.s... |
| Preservative | : 0.15 gm |

Soak the quince seed overnight in two-third of water and strain the mucilage. Melt the stearic acid, cocoa butter and cetyl alcohol. Take glycerine, triethanolamine and water in separate beaker and heated upto 70°C, stir. Add melted fats into the aqueous phase with constant stirring. When the mixture is emulsified, stir the quince seed mucilage into the mixture and continue stirring until cool and smooth.

Add the perfume and preservative previously dissolved in the alcohol. Mix gently.

## f) Vanishing Creams:

Vanishing creams are oil-in-water emulsions with stearic acid or one of its fat like hydrophilic esters as the major emulsified ingredients. They are mainly used to provide fairness to the skin and as a component of make-up to hold face powder and improve its adhesion.

The main ingredients of vanishing creams are excess stearic acid, a soap and water. Soap is prepared *in situ* by the chemical reaction between an alkali and a part (28 – 30%) of stearic acid added. Water used must be strictly purified water otherwise it will have the tendency to invert the emulsion and reduce the stability of the cream by the formation of soaps of divalent ions like calcium and magnesium.

The choice of alkali is an important criteria in preparing vanishing creams. Various alkalis used include potassium hydroxide, sodium hydroxide, potassium carbonate, sodium carbonate, aqueous ammonia, triethanolamine and borax. Of these alkalis, potassium hydroxide is the most suitable because it makes a cream of fine texture and excellent consistency. Sodium hydroxide when used alone makes a hard cream thus it is used in combination with potassium hydroxide. The carbonates are not favoured because they liberate carbon dioxide and render the cream to become spongy. Ammonia is effective but extremely objectionable to handle because of its odour and volatility. Ammonia creams also tend to turn yellow with age. Borax is used, usually in combination with potassium hydroxide or triethanolamine, because it produces a very white emulsion.

Since vanishing creams are o/w type of emulsion, there is possibility of drying out of the cream due to evaporation of water from the external phase of emulsion. To check this, five to ten percent of glycerine and other polyols are added to the creams as humectants.

Vanishing creams may also be prepared by using few other emulsifying agents like triethanolamine soap, amino glycol soap or glyceryl monostearate. But such creams do not produce luster as it has been produced in the creams made from potash alkali and stearic acid.

The lustre or pearliness reflects in the vanishing cream on standing for about two weeks because of the formation of minute crystals of stearic acid. Being an oil-in-water emulsion, it must possess a suitable preservative like parabens.

| Formula – I: Vanishing Cream | |
|---|---|
| Stearic acid | : 25 gm |
| Water | : 64 ml |
| Glycerine | : 10 ml |
| Potassium hydroxide | : 0.8 gm |
| Methyl parahydroxybenzoate | : 0.2 gm |
| Perfume | : ...q.s... |

Melt the stearic acid in a beaker. Dissolve potassium hydroxide and methyl parahydroxybenzoate in water in a separate beaker and add glycerine to it. Heat the aqueous solution upto 65 - 70°C and add to melted stearic acid with constant stirring. Perfume is added to the emulsified mass when the temperature cools down to 45°C. Mix gently.

# Cosmetics for Skin

| Formula – II: Vanishing Cream | |
|---|---|
| Stearic acid XXX | : 15.8 gm |
| Cetyl alcohol | : 0.5 gm |
| Glycerine | : 5 ml |
| Potassium hydroxide | : 1 gm |
| Methyl parahydroxybenzoate | : 0.2 gm |
| Purified water | : 77.5 ml |
| Perfume | : …q.s… |

Melt stearic acid (triple pressed) and cetyl alcohol in a beaker. Take other ingredients except perfume in a separate beaker. Heat upto 70°C and add the hot aqueous solution to melted fat with constant stirring. Perfume is added to cream when it attains temperature nearly 45°C. Mix gently.

g) **Foundation Creams:**

When certain pigments, particularly titanium dioxide, are milled with vanishing creams, they are then termed as foundation creams. They are applied on face before starting make-up. They provide a foundation or base surface for better applicability of make-up.

| Formula: Foundation Cream | |
|---|---|
| Stearic acid XXX | : 15.8 gm |
| Cetyl alcohol | : 0.5 gm |
| Glycerine | : 5 ml |
| Potassium hydroxide | : 1 gm |
| Titanium dioxide | : 2 gm |
| Methyl paraben | : 0.2 gm |
| Purified water | : 75.5 ml |
| Colour | : …q.s… |
| Perfume | : …q.s… |

The method of preparation is the same as in case of vanishing cream. Titanium dioxide is not added initially during preparation. It is added after the cream is being prepared. It is milled with the finished cream with the help of roller mill.

**h) Liquid Creams:**

These creams are emulsions. They are creamy liquids and often termed as lotions, like hand lotions, foundation lotions, moisturizing lotions etc.

The advantage of these creams as against solid creams are that they may be applied easily and uniformly over large surfaces of the skin, they are more easily absorbed and spread out in very thin layers, thereby eliminating the oily feel, so often experienced by solid creams.

The product stability and the texture including its flow property, whiteness, smoothness, breaking of emulsion etc., depends on the type of emulsifying agents used. Apart from emulsifying agents, other operations which are particularly important are the quantities of water, oil, thickner if used, and order in which these materials are handled.

Other parameters which are usually important in all emulsions include the speed and time of mixer and mixing operation, purity of the raw materials, temperature at which the emulsion is made and the pH of the cream.

Materials which are commonly used to prepare liquid creams include vegetable oils usually peanut oil, mineral oil, lanolin, beeswax, spermaceti, caresin, cetyl alcohol or isopropyl esters of the fatty acids, glycerine or propylene glycol. Preservatives are added since they become necessary to prevent the microbial growth in either phases i.e. aqueous and oily. Methyl and propyl parabens are commonly used preservatives to preserve aqueous and oily phase of emulsion respectively.

## Cosmetics for Skin

**Formula – I: Liquid Cream**

| | |
|---|---|
| Stearic acid XXX | : 4 gm |
| Glycerine | : 10 gm |
| Potassium hydroxide | : 0.5 gm |
| Alcohol | : 5 ml |
| Purified water | : 80 ml |
| Perfume | : …q.s… |

Dissolve alkali in purified water, add glycerine to it and heat it upto 70°C. Melt stearic acid in a separate beaker and then aqueous solution added to it with constant stirring. When emulsified mass cool, add perfume dissolved in alcohol.

**Formula – II: Liquid Cream**

| | |
|---|---|
| Stearic acid XXX | : 3 gm |
| Cetyl alcohol | : 1 gm |
| Glycerine | : 6 ml |
| Triethanolamine | : 0.75 gm |
| Borax | : 0.5 gm |
| Purified water | : 88.25 ml |
| Perfume | : …q.s… |

Melt the stearic acid and cetyl alcohol in a beaker. Take triethanolamine, borax and glycerine and water in a separate beaker and heat upto 70°C. Then add melted wax to it with vigorous stirring. Continue the stirring till the temperature comes down to 45°C and then add the perfume.

**Formula – III: Liquid Cream**

| | |
|---|---|
| Stearic acid | : 4.5 gm |
| Glycerine | : 7 ml |
| Potassium hydroxide | : 0.2 gm |
| Alcohol | : 8 ml |
| Lanolin | : 2 gm |
| Purified water | : 780 ml |
| Perfume | : …q.s… |

# Cosmetics for Skin

Dissolve the alkali in purified water. Add glycerine and heat to 70°C. Melt stearic acid and lanolin in a separate beaker. Add aqueous phase to the melted fats with constant stirring. When cool add perfume dissolved in alcohol.

### i) Miscellaneous Creams:

Miscellaneous creams include acid creams, bleaching creams and astringent creams. These creams are prepared for the specific reason of the skin.

- **Acid Creams:**

The utility of skin creams depends on the pH of the skin. Usually, skin is covered with a coating having pH value of 3 to 5. But depending on the physical conditions, perspiration and sebaceous gland secretions, may be more or less alkaline. Thus, skin treatment must be decided after confirming the skin pH of an individual. If alkaline skin treatment is employed without knowing the pH, it may disturb the protective acid layer of the skin and ultimately breaks down natural protection against bacterial invasion of the skin and allows microbial growth. But on the other hand, creams with acid reactions are employed, they promote protection of the skin.

Acid creams can be prepared by the addition of mild acids like citric acid, tartaric acid, malic acid, lactic acid or phosphoric acid, in the suitable cream formula. Here, precaution is taken in the selection of emulsifying agents which might have lost their emulsifying property due to acids present in the formula.

| Formula: Acid Cream | |
|---|---|
| Acid emulsifying agent (Fatty alcohol type) | : 10 gm |
| Stearyl alcohol | : 3.5 gm |
| Glycerine | : 7 ml |
| Purified water | : 78.8 ml |
| Citric acid | : 0.2 gm |
| Perfume | : ...q.s... |

Acid emulsifying agent is partially phosphated cetyl/stearyl alcohol, which is found most suitable for acid creams. The above preparation is prepared by dissolving citric acid in

# Cosmetics for Skin

purified water and add glycerine to it, heat it upto 70°C. Melt emulsifying agent and stearyl alcohol in a separate beaker and then aqueous solution is added to it with constant stirring. When cool, add perfume.

- **Bleaching Creams:**

Bleaching creams are used to bleach the skin. Many bleaching agents like hydrogen peroxide and other peroxides, sodium perborate, lactic acid, citric acid, bismuth subnitrate etc. are added to the creamy base for this purpose.

| Formula: Bleaching Cream | |
|---|---|
| Petrolatum | : 40 gm |
| Spermaceti | : 14 gm |
| Mineral oil | : 27 ml |
| Lanolin | : 4 gm |
| Glycerine | : 4 ml |
| Hydrogen peroxide | : 3 ml |
| Lactic acid | : 3.5 gm |
| Acetic acid | : 0.4 ml |
| Purified water | : 3 ml |
| Methyl paraben | : 0.1 gm |
| Perfume | : ...q.s... |

Mix the glycerine with purified water and dissolve methyl paraben, lactic acid and acetic acid in one beaker. Melt the spermaceti, lanolin and petrolatum in another beaker and then add the mineral oil, mix thoroughly. Add acidic solution to melted oily phase with constant stirring. When cool add hydrogen peroxide and perfume. Continue mixing to obtain a uniformly mixed cream.

The users are directed to use the cream with precaution as it is a very strong bleaching cream.

- **Astringent Creams:**

Astringent creams are used to correct excessive oiliness of the skin. They control this by reducing the permeability of the cell membrane. The astringent action is accompanied by contraction and wrinkling of the tissue and by bleaching. They precipitate proteins and cause slight inflammation and reddening of the skin which makes the skin surface opening less conspicuous.

The principal astringents are salts of aluminium, zinc, manganese, iron and bismuth. Tannins or related polyphenolic compounds are also used as astringents.

| Formula: Astringent Cream | |
|---|---|
| Alum | : 0.2 gm |
| Zinc sulphate | : 0.2 gm |
| Glycerine | : 15.5 ml |
| Pulverized gum acacia | : 2 gm |
| White beeswax | : 15 gm |
| Cocoa butter | : 2 gm |
| Purified water | : 64 ml |
| Preservative | : 0.1 gm |
| Perfume | : ...q.s... |

Dissolve zinc sulphate and alum in glycerine, preservative together with an equal amount of water by means of heat. Dissolve the gum acacia in the remainder of the water, strain and heat the mixture. Melt the beeswax and cocoa butter and add the acacia mucilage to it with rapid agitation. Then add alum, zinc sulphate mixture with constant stirring. When cool, add perfume.

**Lotion Preparations:**

Lotions are very popular in the field of cosmetics. They are liquid applications mainly for the skin and to produce a beautifying effect. The lotion must provide emollient as well as soothing effect.

In our previous discussion we described liquid creams as lotions since they are emulsions of fatty and oily materials. But here, lotions might be the liquid preparations containing gums and thin liquid preparations made without gums.

# Cosmetics for Skin

Materials which are generally used for these types of lotions include water, glycerine and other humectants, alcohols, gums and similar thickeners, astringents, antiseptics, cooling agents and miscellaneous other ingredients.

a) **Hand Lotions:**

Hand lotions are prepared to protect hands which receive most of the wear and tear. They are quite useful for persons washing dish, cleaning house and other such activities which tend to turn skin rough. Thus the main function of hand lotions is to soothe and soften roughened hands.

These are non-greasy liquid products, thus applied many times during the day. This characteristics of these lotions makes them popular as against over other oily lotions.

| Formula: Tragacanth Hand Lotion | |
|---|---|
| Tragacanth | : 1.25 gm |
| Purified water | : 85 ml |
| Glycerine | : 6 ml |
| Borax | : 1.25 gm |
| Tincture benzoin | : 0.3 ml |
| Alcohol | : 3 ml |
| Distilled witch hazel | : 2.7 ml |
| Perfume | : ...q.s... |

Make a mucilage of gum tragacanth with 50 parts of purified water. Make up tincture benzoin and strained. Dissolve borax in rest of the water, add glycerine and distilled witch hazel, heat upto 60 - 70°C. Add mucilage, then alcohol in which the perfume has been dissolved. While stirring, add the tincture. Mix well, strain and fill when cool.

b) **Skin Toning Lotions:**

Now – a – days skin toning lotions are very much popular and are known as skin freshners. They are usually limpid liquids, with weakly astringent, stimulating and antiseptic properties. They are employed to freshen the skin and to remove residual traces of make up.

# Cosmetics for Skin

It is very simple to formulate skin tonning lotions by dissolving the ingredients in the water, alcohol and suitable liquids and then filter. To maintain the clearity of the liquid, filter aids like talc, magnesia etc. are added. They can be made coloured by using approved water soluble colours.

| Formula – I: Skin Toning Lotions | |
|---|---|
| Boric acid | : 1 gm |
| Witch hazel | : 15 ml |
| Rose water | : 15 ml |
| Alcohol | : 8 ml |
| Orange flower water | : 61 ml |

Warm the witch hazel and dissolve the boric acid in it. Mix the rest of the ingredients with the orange flower water and add the boric acid solution, mix, keep it for a week and filter using suitable filter aid (talc).

| Formula – II: Skin Toning Lotion | |
|---|---|
| Menthol | : 0.05 gm |
| Glycerine | : 5 ml |
| Alcohol | : 5 ml |
| Boric acid | : 2 gm |
| Bay rum | : 10 ml |
| Purified water | : 77.7 ml |
| Perfume | : …q.s… |

Dissolve the menthol in alcohol in one beaker and boric acid in sufficient warm water. Mix the rest of the water with bay rum. Add the menthol solution to the rum solution. Mix it. Add boric acid solution and glycerine to the menthol solution. Finally, add the perfume mixed with a little talc (sterilized), mix and keep the mixture for at least a week and then filter.

## Cosmetics for Skin

### c) Astringent Lotions:

As described in astringent creams, lotions are also intended to correct excessive oiliness and also to hike coarse pores of the skin. The proper treatment of oiliness is to use an astringent cream at night and as an astringent lotion in the morning before the application of face powder.

Astringents are divided into two classes; true astringents and pseudo-astringents. True astringents precipitate proteins, e.g. tannates and aluminium ion. Pseudo astringents produce physiological effects without combining with proteins, e.g. cold water when applied to the skin is widely recognized as having an astringent effect. Similarly, alcohol, evaporates more quickly, can act as an efficient astringent.

Many astringents are used to make lotions like tannic acid, aluminium sulphate or chloride, zinc oxide, etc.

| Formula – I: Astringent Lotion | |
|---|---|
| Alum | : 0.75 gm |
| Zinc sulphate | : 0.1 gm |
| Glycerine | : 8 ml |
| Alcohol | : 12 ml |
| Purified water | : 78.65 ml |
| Perfume | : ...q.s... |

Dissolve the alum in little part of purified water in one beaker. Add zinc sulphate in the glycerine in another beaker, add remainder of purified water. Add the alum solution and alcohol to the zinc sulphate solution. Allow to stand for 48 hours and then filter.

| Formula – II: Astringent Lotion | |
|---|---|
| Zinc phenol sulphonate | : 0.75 gm |
| Camphor | : 0.5 gm |
| Menthol | : 0.5 gm |
| Perfume | : ...q.s... |
| Alcohol | : 12 ml |
| Witch hazel | : 85.8 ml |

# Cosmetics for Skin

Dissolve camphor, menthol and perfume in alcohol in one beaker. Dissolve zinc phenol sulphonates in witch hazel. Then add witch hazel solution to alcoholic solution with constant stirring. Allow the solution to keep for 24 hours and then filter.

### d) Bleaching and Freckle Lotions:

In the world of cosmetic bleaching creams and lotions are gaining the popularity since they are instantly used to make the skin fair. It is not a permanent change of the skin but for a short period. True bleaching of skin colour is impossible as the pigmentation cells of skin lie in the basal layer of the epidermis and no skin preparation can reach to the pigments. Bleaching preparations act on surface pigmentation chemically and lighten the skin. Sometimes, surface irritants cause the skin to flake off and expose the fresh lighter coloured outer layer of the skin or the cornium.

Many ingredients act chemically as bleaching agents include, lactic acid, acetic acid, citric acid, hydrogen and metallic peroxides, sodium and zinc perborate, potassium chlorate, lemon juice, bismuth subnitrate etc.

Some skin irritants can also be used for bleaching of the skin include, ammoniated mercury, formaldehyde, salicylic acid and zinc sulphocarbolate etc.

**Formula – I: Bleaching Lotion**

| | |
|---|---|
| Hydrogen peroxide | : 60 ml |
| Distilled water | : 40 ml |

Mix the two ingredients. Make fresh for better result.

**Formula – II: Bleaching Lotion**

| | |
|---|---|
| Lactic acid | : 2 gm |
| Acetic acid | : 2 ml |
| Citric acid | : 3 gm |
| Glycerine | : 10 ml |
| Alcohol | : 10 ml |
| Purified water | : 72.5 ml |
| Perfume | : ...q.s... |

Dissolve the citric acid in the water and the acetic acid in the glycerine. Mix the two solutions and add lactic acid. Add perfume already dissolved in alcohol. Keep the preparation overnight and filter.

It is a strong preparation. A cold cream is recommended after its use.

| Formula – III: Freckle Lotion | |
|---|---|
| Acetic acid | : 3 ml |
| Concentrated lemon juice | : 10 ml |
| Glycerine | : 8 ml |
| Purified water | : 68.5 ml |
| Alcohol | : 10 ml |
| Perfume | : …q.s… |

Dissolve the concentrated lemon juice and the acetic acid in the water. Add perfume dissolved in the alcohol, add glycerine and add this solution to the lemon juice solution. Mix and filter.

e) **After Shave Lotions:**

This particular lotion is employed by the men after shaving to provide emollient effect, astringent effect, softening of beard and antiseptic effect in case of razor cuts. They are very much liked by their cooling and refreshing feeling after application, which are obtained by the addition of ingredients like capsicum or cantharides and high content of alcohol. The most popular perfumes used lilac, lavender, bay rum etc.

| Formula: After Shave Lotion | |
|---|---|
| Boric acid | : 2 gm |
| Menthol | : 0.05 gm |
| Glycerine | : 2 ml |
| Alcohol | : 8 ml |
| Witch hazel | : 87.45 ml |
| Perfume | : …q.s… |

Dissolve boric acid in witch hazel. Add glycerine into it. Menthol and perfume are dissolved in alcohol in a separate beaker. Add alcoholic solution slowly to aqueous solution with constant stirring. Filter it.

# Cosmetics for Skin

**Miscellaneous Preparations:**

Few miscellaneous preparations which are used on skin include deodorants, bathing preparations, make-up preparations and suntan preparations. These preparations are discussed in the subsequent sub sections.

**a) Deodorants:**

There is a noticeable problem of body odour from men and women. Everyone wants to get rid of himself from the objectionable body odour. This problem cannot be eliminated by taking frequent baths, because perspiration, being continuous and deposited slowly on the skin surface, which may become malodorous in a period of four to six hours after bath.

To correct the body malodorous odour, there are two methods; (1) Use of deodorants and (2) Use of antiperspirants.

Since, antiperspirants are rather drugs instead of cosmetics, they will not be dealt here.

There are two types of deodorants, one is employed to deodorize perspiration without restricting its flow and the other one is employed to deodorize and prevent decomposition through bacteria inhibiting action.

Deodorants may be liquids, pastes, powders, compacts and sticks. Before compounding a deodorant, it is required to decide what type of deodorant it shall be? Secondly to determine its specific use. Usually deodorants are used for the arms pits, but some may be used for deodorizing sanitary napkins. It is quite obvious that a deodorant in the latter use, should not be an astringent. Thus, a deodorant may be antiseptic, or it may be an astringent, depending on its use.

Among the materials used are boric acid, benzoic acid, oxyquinoline sulphate, formaldehyde, zinc salicylate, zinc sulphocarbolates, aluminium acetate, aluminium chloride, alum etc. As no one material possesses all properties for an effective deodorant hence it becomes necessary to utilize two or more to produce a desired product.

Oxyquinoline sulphate is said to be an excellent ingredients because it is not only a powerful antiseptic but it is an excellent deodorant besides being non-toxic and non-irritating properties.

# Cosmetics for Skin

| Formula – I: Deodorant Liquid | |
|---|---|
| Oxyquinoline sulphate | : 2 gm |
| Aluminium chloride | : 14 gm |
| Magnesium sulphate | : 7 gm |
| Alcohol | : 4 ml |
| Purified water | : 72.5 ml |
| Perfume | : …q.s… |

Mix all the three salts in purified water and then add perfume dissolved in alcohol.

| Formula – II: Deodorant Paste | |
|---|---|
| Petrolatum | : 56.3 gm |
| Zinc oxide | : 20 gm |
| Benzoic acid | : 5 gm |
| Propyl paraben | : 0.2 gm |
| Hydrogenated vegetable oil | : 18 ml |
| Perfume | : …q.s… |

Melt and mix all ingredients.

| Formula – III: Deodorant Powder | |
|---|---|
| Purified zinc peroxide | : 40 gm |
| Boric acid | : 18 gm |
| Talc | : 41.5 gm |
| Perfume | : …q.s… |

Mix all ingredients in ascending order, sift them and add perfume.

# Cosmetics for Skin

| Formula – IV: Deodorant Cream | |
|---|---|
| Glyceryl monostearate | : 15 gm |
| Titanium oxide | : 1 gm |
| Petrolatum | : 4 gm |
| Beeswax | : 2 gm |
| Formaldehyde (40%) | : 1 ml |
| Purified water | : 77 ml |

Take all ingredients except formaldehyde in a beaker, heat on water bath. When a uniform mixture is formed, stop heating and stir the mixture until a smooth cream is formed. Add formaldehyde solution when cool (45°C). Stir to obtain uniform cream.

**b) Bathing preparations:**

In modern age, bath preparations are becoming popular in high societies. The use of these preparations came into mind when bathtubs were introduced. As such, if we define bathing, which is nothing but the cleaning of whole body either simply by water or water along with the soap. But this simple bathing operation is being thought to be improved so as to make this operation more enjoyable in incense atmosphere.

Many cosmetologists paid attention towards this new era and developed some of the bathing beauty preparations for the following functions:

i) To cleanse the skin.
ii) To perfume the bath.
iii) To soften the water.
iv) To form bubbles or foam in the bath water.
v) To leave the skin rejuvenated with cool feeling.

These preparations are classified as Bath soaps, bath salts (water softeners), bath oils (perfumed media), surface active agents (bubble baths) and dusting or after bath powders.

Bath soaps are commonly used as cleansers of the body. They are different from ordinary toilet soap in having more proportions of tallow soap base suitable perfumed and coloured to meet consumers appeal. Usually bath soap cake is bigger than the toilet soap cake. As with certain toilet soaps, other fats and oils than tallow and coconut oil enter the

# Cosmetics for Skin

bath soap fat charge to assign presumed special quality and value to them. Thus, palm oil and olive oil soaps are featured as superior soaps for bathing.

Bath salts form another type of bathing preparations which contain wetting agents and alkalies to improve the cleansing property. The main purpose of bath salts is to soften the bath water, scent the water, build up its cleansing power and prevent the problem of itching to which certain individuals are sensitive.

Now-a-days, number of chemicals are available for making bath salts. Few of them include sodium sesquicarbonate, borax and other phosphates like trisodium phosphate, sodium hexametaphosphate and tetra sodium pyrophosphate. These salts possess good detergent as well as water softening property.

Both oils comprise another type of bath preparations which are solely employed to perfume the bathing water. They are concentrated products of scents dissolved in various solvents like water miscible mineral oil, isopropyl alcohol, solvent esters and alcohol. Emulsifying agents are also added to these preparations to assure a better dispersion of perfume throughout the water.

Bubble baths preparations are employed to generate lot of foam in the bathtub. They contain mainly of surface active or wetting agents serving the purpose of detergency and generating foam.

Dusting and after bath powders are also categorized under bathing preparations.

| Formula – I: Bath Salts | |
|---|---|
| Sodium sesquicarbonate | : 99 gm |
| Perfume and colour | : …q.s… |

Mix the ingredients by spraying perfume and colour on the sodium sesquicarbonate salt in the mixer.

| Formula – II: Bath Oil | |
|---|---|
| Equ de cologne compound | : 5 gm |
| Sulphonated olive oil | : 95 ml |

Mix the two ingredients.

# Cosmetics for Skin

| Formula – III: Liquid Bubble Bath | |
|---|---|
| Alkyl aryl sulphate | : 5 gm |
| Distilled water | : 95 ml |

Dissolve alkyl aryl sulphate in distilled water with very slow stirring. Vigorous stirring is avoided to avoid generation of foam.

### c) Make-up preparations:

Make up preparations are greatly employed in enhancing the personal appearance by tinting skin and hair. For any make up preparation to be applied on the skin, a base of foundation cream is applied. Initially vanishing cream was used as foundation cream for the purpose to complement the use of face powders and other make up preparations. Vanishing cream forms translucent flexible film of soap stearic acid-glycerine to which the make up preparations adhere more readily than to the bare skin. But in many cases, this film is not opaque enough, thus, the use of foundation cream augmented which is vanishing cream with 5 – 50% pigments providing opacity.

Other make-up preparations, which are discussed here are rouges, lipsticks, mascara and eye shadow.

### i) Rouges:

These are very important preparations of a make-up box. Rouges are specially applied on the cheeks for enhancing the entire look of the face. They impart sparked touch and stimulate the freshness of the skin. They are prepared by the mixtures of fats, oils and waxes, suitably coloured. They are available in various forms like paste, cream and dry solid.

| Formula – I: Paste Rouge | |
|---|---|
| Spermaceti | : 6.5 gm |
| Cetyl alcohol | : 2.5 gm |
| Cocoa butter | : 2.5 gm |
| White beeswax | : 2.5 gm |
| White petrolatum | : 77 gm |
| Cosmetic lake colour | : 8 gm |

# Cosmetics for Skin

| Preservative | : 0.1 ml |
| Perfume | : …q.s… |

Melt all the waxes and other fatty material, mix and mill. Add colour and perfume and mill to get homogeneous product.

| **Formula – II: Vanishing Cream type Rouge** | |
|---|---|
| Stearic acid XXX | : 18 gm |
| Cetyl alcohol | : 4 gm |
| Glycerine | : 9 ml |
| Water | : 60.1 ml |
| Potassium hydroxide (85%) | : 0.6 gm |
| Cosmetic lake colour | : 8 gm |
| Perfume | : …q.s… |

Follow the method of preparation as in case of vanishing cream. Add colour and perfume in the cream, mill thoroughly to get uniform product.

## ii) Mascara:

Mascara is a dark pigmented preparation used for eyelashes to render curved upward at the end. This improves the beauty of eyes and also provides dark colour to the eyelashes. There are few precautions which are to be taken during the preparation of mascara since it is to be applied to the most sensitive part of the body. They include:

- Materials used must be non-toxic and non-irritating to the eyes.
- They should not run and causes eyelashes to stick together after applications.
- The colour must be harmless and intense in shade.

Various colour shades are used in mascara like lamp black, brown shade or synthetic ochre with or without the addition of traces of lampblack. As a rule mascara is applied with a special brush.

Mascara are prepared in three forms, e.g. liquid, cream and cake. Liquid mascara are suspension of colouring matter, usually in a light mucilaginous vehicle. Gum acacia,

# Cosmetics for Skin

tragacanth, karaya and gelatin are useful for mucilage. Gelatin increases the ability of the mascara to cling to the lashes.

In cream type of mascara, an emulsion prepared by glyceryl monostearate and water combined with suitable colour is effective.

The most convenient and popular type of mascara is the cake type, which is prepared by milling toilet soap, sometimes with beeswax and petrolatum along with proper colour.

| Formula – I: Cream Mascara | |
|---|---|
| Glyceryl monostearate | : 10 gm |
| Triethanolamine | : 3 gm |
| Stearic acid | : 17 gm |
| Petrolatum | : 18 gm |
| Gelatin | : 2 gm |
| Purified water | : 17 ml |
| Beeswax | : 25 gm |
| Prepared lampblack | : 8 gm |

Soak the gelatin in hot water. Melt the beeswax, stearic acid, petrolatum and glyceryl monostearate, stir in the lampblack thoroughly. Add triethanolamine to the soaked gelatin and then add the mixture to the melted mass. Stir continuously to get a uniform creamy mascara.

**iii) Eye shadows:**

Eye shadows are the preparations used to impart background shadow to the eyes and are applied to the eyelids and around the eyes to enhance their brilliance. The common colours used in eye shadows are blue, green, white gold and silver. They are also available in creams sticks and lose powder forms. They are applied with the help of fine camel brush.

| Formula: Eye Shadow Blue | |
|---|---|
| White beeswax | : 3 gm |
| Spermaceti | : 3.75 gm |
| Lanolin | : 3.5 gm |
| White petrolatum | : 43.65 gm |

# Cosmetics for Skin

| Ultramarine | : 15 gm |
| Zinc oxide | : 30.85 gm |
| Perfume | : ...q.s... |

Mix the colour with zinc oxide and then white petrolatum is added to it. Mill through ointment mill. Melt the beeswax, spermaceti and lanolin. Add the colour base and perfume. Mill the final mixture to obtain uniform product.

### iv) Eyebrow pencils:

Eyebrow pencils are high wax containing hard crayons for darkening the eyebrows and to impart pseudogrowth of the eyebrows when none is evident, usually they contain black colour. They can be easily sharpended to apply exactly on the eyebrows.

| **Formula: Eyebrow Pencils** | |
|---|---|
| Yellow wax | : 12 gm |
| Paraffin wax | : 28 gm |
| Cocoa butter | : 32 gm |
| Petrolatum | : 18 gm |
| Carbon black | : 10 gm |

Melt and mix in mill. Mould in pencil moulds.

### v) Lipsticks:

Women are very much conscious to improve the beauty of their lips which stand important position in enhancing their personality. This is the reason why the consumption of lipsticks is continuously increasing. The important criteria to choose the lipsticks is their colour shades. Some like natural colour lipsticks just to give natural shining to the lips and other may like bright colours.

The raw materials to prepare lipsticks include fats, oils and waxes, dyes, perfume oils and some other additive to provide special properties.

# Cosmetics for Skin

Various fats, oils and waxes are used which include castor oil, butyl stearate, undecylic acid, stearyl alcohol, oleyl alcohol, cocoa butter, beeswax, ozokerite, carnauba wax, spermaceti, cetyl alcohol, mineral oil, petrolatum, paraffin, glyceryl monostearate etc.

A good quality lipstick must have the following characteristics:

It should:

- Be non-toxic, non-irritating and free from gritty particles,
- Be easy to apply on the lips and also to remove,
- Have good and shiny appearance,
- Be firm physically, should not be broken during application,
- Have good spreadability, the colour must remain for longer period.

| Formula: Lipstick |         |
|---|---|
| White beeswax | : 35 gm |
| Cetyl alcohol | : 10 gm |
| Seasame oil | : 19 ml |
| Castor oil | : 30 ml |
| Tetrabromofluorescein | : 4 gm |
| Perfume | : …q.s… |

Dissolve tetrabromofluorescein in castor oil. Melt white beeswax, cetyl alcohol and then add seasame oil. Add both the mixtures and add perfume. Mix and mill thoroughly to get uniform mass. Fill the mass into the cavities of the mould.

# 3. COSMETICS FOR HAIR AND SHAVING MEDIA

**Cosmetics for Hair and Shaving Media:**

Cosmetics for hair and shaving media are further classified as follows:

a) Shampoos
b) Scalp and dandruff tonics
c) Brilliantines and hair dressings
d) Hair waving preparations
e) Depilatories
f) Pre-shaving lotions
g) Shaving media

**a) Shampoos:**

Now-a-days, shampoos are commonest preparations to be used on hair for cleaning and make them manageable and lustrous. They contain surface active agents for the purpose of cleaning, i.e. removal of grease, dirt and debris from the hair and scalp without showing any untowards effects on hair, scalp and other parts of the body.

Shampoos are supposed to leave good fragrance in hair after cleaning and turn hair soft, silky and lustrous, so that they can be easily managed. A good shampoo possesses the following qualities:

- It should perform its function in small amount.
- It should be effective in removing the dirt and debris from the hair and scalp.
- It should be non-toxic, non-irritant to the skin and eyes.
- It should able to build foam in soft as well as hard water.
- It should be easily washable with water.
- It should leave fragrance in hair after washing.
- It should turn hair soft, silky and lustrous.
- It should make the hair easily manageable.

Shampoos are prepared by two ways, i.e. using synthetic detergents or using soaps.

# Cosmetics for Hair and Shaving Media

Synthetic detergent based shampoos are very much popular. They are available in liquid, emulsion, paste, gel or powder forms suitably coloured and perfumed. These shampoos must comply with the requirements like; it should have pH 5 to 9. It should be clear or transparent if liquid, it should not have any sign of breaking of phases, if emulsion, it should be free from any agglomerated particles if paste; it should have free flowing property if powder form. Colours used must be confirmed with the provisions of relevant Indian Standard subject to the provisions of Schedule Q of the Drugs and Cosmetics Act and Rules.

Ingredients required to manufacture synthetic detergent based shampoos are summarised in following table:

**Table: Examples of ingredients used in the formulation of synthetic detergent based shampoos**

| | |
|---|---|
| Detergents | - Sodium lauryl sulphate<br>- Alkyl benzene polyoxyethyl sulphonates<br>- Sodium lauryl sarcosinate<br>- Triethanolamine lauryl sulphate<br>- Triethanolamine alkyl sulphate |
| Foam stabilizers | - Ethanolamides<br>- Isopropanolamides of fatty acids<br>- Amine oxides |
| Chelating agents | - Sodium polyphosphates<br>- Sodium salts of EDTA |
| Solubilizing agents | - Urea<br>- Alcohol<br>- Glycols<br>- Surfactants |
| Preservatives | - Alcohols<br>- Methyl and propyl parabens |
| Opacifying agents | - Higher fatty alcohols<br>- Ethylene / propylene glycol stearates |

# Cosmetics for Hair and Shaving Media

|  |  |
|---|---|
|  | - Mono or di-stearates of glycerol |
|  | - Salts of fatty acids |
| Emollients (Conditioning agents) | - Lanolin and its derivatives |
|  | - Glycerol esters |
|  | - Fatty alcohols |
| Thickening agents | - Methyl cellulose |
|  | - Sodium CMC |
|  | - Sodium alginate |
|  | - Polyvinyl alcohol |
|  | - Ethyl cellulose |
|  | - Sodium or potassium chloride |
| Antidandruff agents | - Hexachlorophene |
|  | - Selenium sulphide |
|  | - Selenium disulphide |
| Others | - Colours |
|  | - Perfumes |

All these shampoo additives perform their functions like;

i) **Detergents:** They clean the hair, remove dirt and debris from hair and scalp. They have removed the disadvantages of hard water in which soaps do not give foam.

ii) **Foam stabilizers:** They increase the quality, volume and stability of the foam. They also enhance viscosity and leave slight conditioning effect.

iii) **Chelating agents:** They are added to prevent the formation of lime soap due to the presence of hard water.

iv) **Solubilizing agents:** They are added to solubilize poorly soluble ingredients and hence to avoid and haziness in the shampoo.

v) **Preservatives:** They are added to preserve shampoo from microbial growth.

vi) **Opacifying agents:** They are added to turn shampoo opaque.

vii) **Emollients:** They are added to improve the texture of the hair and to render them manageable, lustrous and silky.

## Cosmetics for Hair and Shaving Media

viii) **Thickening agents:** They are added to enhance the viscosity of the shampoos. Their quantity is adjusted to provide desired consistency of the preparation.

ix) **Antidandruff agents:** They are used to reduce dandruff from the hair.

x) **Other additives:** They are suitable colours and perfumes, added to shampoos to improve their cosmetic appeal.

Soap based shampoos contain soaps which are the salts of higher fatty acids. Soaps are obtained by saponifying the natural animal and vegetable fats and oils with alkalis like sodium or potassium hydroxides. Soap based shampoos should be clear liquid, free from sediment and suitably coloured and perfumed. They are formulated by using all the additives of detergent based shampoos.

| Formula - I: Coconut Oil Shampoo (Soap Based) | |
|---|---|
| Coconut oil | : 10 ml |
| Potassium hydroxide (85%) | : 5.38 gm |
| Sodium hydroxide (95%) | : 0.5 gm |
| Glycerine | : 13 ml |
| Oleic acid | : 14 gm |
| Water | : 56.72 ml |
| Perfume | : ...q.s... |

Dissolve potassium hydroxide in one-third of the water. Heat coconut oil on water bath and add the alkali solution in a thin stream with continuous stirring until saponified. Allow the coconut soap to become cold, stand overnight. Mix glycerine with half of the remaining water and bring it to boil, then add coconut soap in small portions and stir until dissolved. Dissolve the sodium hydroxide in the rest of the water and add to the soap solution immediately after the coconut soap has dissolved. Add the oleic acid and stir slowly until completely saponified, then perfume. Keep the product for few days, chill to 32°C and then filter.

# Cosmetics for Hair and Shaving Media

| Formula - II: Cream Shampoo (Detergent Based) | |
|---|---|
| Sodium lauryl sulphate (SLS) | : 15 gm |
| Stearic acid | : 13 gm |
| Lanolin | : 0.5 gm |
| Caustic soda | : 2 gm |
| Cetyl alcohol | : 1 gm |
| Purified water | : 68.5 ml |
| Colour | : …q.s… |
| Perfume | : …q.s… |

Melt stearic acid, lanolin and cetyl alcohol in one beaker and dissolve sodium lauryl sulphate in half of the purified water and caustic soda in the another part of water. Add alkali solution to the melted mass with constant stirring and then the solution of sodium lauryl sulphate is added with gentle stirring. Vigorous stirring is avoided while the addition of SLS solution. When the mixture cools down, add the colour and perfume.

**b) Scalp and dandruff tonics:**

Although the name of these preparations are designated as 'tonic' but it is misleading, since, no external preparation can stimulate hair growth. Still the word 'tonic' persist in the mind of people inspite of technical mistake.

These preparations have been employed for dry scalps and for oily scalps. Those for dry scalps are stimulating the flow of the sebaceous glands. Those for oily scalps are correcting the oily conditions and are usually alkaline in reaction. Simply, because of these functions, they are falsely named as 'tonic'.

| Formula: Hair Tonic | |
|---|---|
| Salicylic acid | : 0.2 gm |
| Fowler's solution | : 10 ml |
| Alcohol | : 30 ml |
| Glycerine | : 5 ml |
| Purified water | : 54 ml |
| Perfume | : …q.s… |

Dissolve salicylic acid in alcohol, add the perfume. Add other ingredients and mix, filter it.

### c) Brilliantines and hair dressings:

Brilliantines are employed to impart luster to the hair and also keeping them in the proper place. They have to be applied to the dry hair after it has been waved. They are available in liquid form or viscous form. Liquid form is liked by women because of ease of application on their long hair while men like viscous creamy form.

| Formula - I: Liquid Brilliantine | |
|---|---|
| Olive oil | : 45 ml |
| Sweet almond oil | : 43.95 ml |
| Castor oil | : 5 ml |
| Parahydroxy Benzoic acid ester | : 0.05 gm |
| Alcohol | : 5 ml |
| Perfume | : ...q.s... |

Dissolve the parahydroxy benzoic acid ester and the perfume in the alcohol and then mix the almond oil. Mix olive and castor oils and add almond oil mixture to it. Allow to stand for three days and filter.

| Formula - II: Jelly Brilliantine | |
|---|---|
| Spermaceti | : 15 gm |
| Myristic acid | : 6 gm |
| Oleic acid | : 25 gm |
| White mineral oil | : 53 ml |
| Perfume | : ...q.s... |

Melt the spermaceti, myristic acid and oleic acid in one beaker. Heat the white mineral oil separately; then mix the two together thoroughly at the same temperature. Perfume at about 45°C.

Hair straighteners are the preparations which are used to take curl or kink out of the hair and at the same time impart a sheen and perfume to the hair. They are applied on the hair with the help of hard brush which aids in removing the curl of the hair. These preparations contain materials like rosin, gums, paraffin, beeswax and castor oil.

| Formula - I: Hair Straightener | |
|---|---|
| Petrolatum | : 90 gm |
| Rosin | : 8 gm |
| Perfume | : ...q.s... |

Melt the rosin with petrolatum. Stir well. Cool slightly and add perfume at 45°C.

| Formula - II: Gum Type Hair Straightener | |
|---|---|
| Glycerine | : 10 ml |
| Powder soap | : 10 gm |
| 2% Mucilage of gum tragacanth | : 54 ml |
| Beeswax | : 25 gm |
| Methyl parahydroxy benzoate | : 0.1 ml |
| Perfume | : ...q.s... |

Melt the wax. Mix glycerine, soap, perfume and preservative with the mucilage. Add the latter mixture to the molten wax and then mix well.

**d) Hair waving preparations:**

These preparations are used to curl or wave the hair. Such products are becoming very much popular in beauty parlours where proper treatment is given to hair for curling them. Hair curl mechanically because there is a great strain along the length of one side of the hair shaft than the other. It there is increase in strain on one side, the hair turn to curl.

To curl or wave hair, they are to be soften and stretched so as to take the proper wave. In beauty parlours soft hair are stretched on rolling them on heat rod so as to cause an unequal strain on one side and then permitting the hair to cool. The hair, thus waved.

# Cosmetics for Hair and Shaving Media

In order to assist the hair curling, various preparations like; curling concentrated powders, permanent wave fluids and hair wave liquids are used.

Material used to prepare these preparations are mucilage of a gum like gum karaya or gum tragacanth with borax or alkali carbonates. Some preparations exclude gums and only contain alkalis like; mixtures of sodium carbonate and sodium bicarbonate. Other bases like; ammonia salts, triethanolamine, trisodium phosphate and tetrasodium pyrophosphate are also used frequently in permanent hair waving preparation. Other supporting materials may be alcohol, glycerine, glycols, lanolin, surface active agents, soaps, sulphonated oils, lanolin and its derivatives, lecithin and certain oils and fatty acids are added to the various preparations.

| Formula - I: Permanent Wave Solution | |
|---|---|
| Ammonium carbonate | : 2 gm |
| Potassium carbonate | : 1.2 gm |
| Potassium sulphite | : 2.5 gm |
| Ammonium hydroxide | : 3.3 gm |
| Sulphonated castor oil | : 1 ml |
| Purified water | : 90 ml |

Dissolve the first four ingredients in purified water, add oil and mix well.

| Formula - II: Karaya Curling Liquid | |
|---|---|
| Gum karaya | : 2 gm |
| Water | : 90.5 ml |
| Methyl paraben | : 0.25 gm |
| Alcohol | : 7 ml |
| Perfume | : ...q.s... |

Mix the gum and half the alcohol and stir the mixture into the water. Strain if necessary. Add the perfume and preservative dissolved in the rest of the alcohol.

# Cosmetics for Hair and Shaving Media

### e) Depilatories:

These preparations are employed for temporarily removing any undesired hair above the outer surface of the skin. Women are the main user of such type of the preparation for removing their unwanted hair of the skin. The action of depilatories is to dissolve the hair. Initially, it is softened, swelled and dispersed by the action of the chemical. These chemicals may have irritating effect on the epidermis if applied and remained on the skin for long time. Thus, the preparations must be so formulated as to complete their reaction in not more than five minutes. After the action has been completed, depilatories must be washed properly with soapy water and then skin is nourished with cold cream. It is necessary to make aware of the users about the proper use of depilatories, otherwise they may create some problems related with the skin. To ensure the safety, the user should be advised to do the sensitivity test on a part of her arm which is devoid of hair, by applying a little depilatory and leaving it on for about five minutes. If the subject finds sensitivity towards the depilatory, she must not use it.

Chemical substances widely used to prepare these preparations are barium sulphide, sodium and potassium sulphides. Other chemicals like tin salts, calcium thioglycerol and calcium thioglycollate are also used. The materials for the carrier are corn starch, talc, titanium dioxide, terra alba, barium sulphate and zinc oxide. Pulverized soap is added to the formulation as a binding agent. It is very difficult to choose a perfect perfume owing to the unpleasant odour of depilatories. However, aromatic alcohols, ketones, ionones, anise, safrol and rose oils are used alone or in combination.

| Formula: Depilatory Powder | |
|---|---|
| Titanium dioxide | : 28 gm |
| Barium sulphide | : 30 gm |
| Wheat starch | : 40 gm |
| Perfume | : ...q.s... |

Sift the titanium dioxide, barium sulphide and wheat starch. Mix all the powders and the perfume in ascending order. Mix the mixture for half an hour.

# Cosmetics for Hair and Shaving Media

### f) Pre-shaving lotions:

Pre-shaving lotions are designed to make beard soft before applying electric razor, safety razor or any other razor. This results in the smooth and close shave without irritation. If razor is applied on the dry skin, it will result in the shaving with irritation or might have few small cuts on the skin. Thus a beard softner is designed to have such type of ingredients which do not only soften hair but help to allay irritation. Sodium cholate which appears quite frequently among the ingredients of beard softner preparations. These preparations are available in lotions as well as cream forms.

| Formula: Pre-Shaving Lotion | |
|---|---|
| Sodium cholate | : 0.35 gm |
| Sodium lauryl sulphate | : 3 gm |
| Glycerine | : 8 ml |
| Purified water | : 88.15 ml |
| Perfume | : …q.s… |

Dissolve the sodium cholate and sodium lauryl sulphate in a mixture of the glycerine and an equal quantity of water. Heat to 60° - 70°C. When solution is affected add remainder of the water and perfume. Keep the solution for a week and filter.

### g) Shaving media:

Shaving media serve the purpose of removing unsightly hair particularly from men's faces or also from the legs, under arms and other conspicuous places of the women. These media include brushless shaving media, lather creams and shaving soaps.

Brushless shaving creams are most popular shaving media because of their convenience and more comfort in shaving. They require no brush for application, occupy less space in travelling shaving kit and may be applied to the face more rapidly. They provide more comfortable shave because they soften the beard facilitating shaving operation. They leave the face with a thin coating of the oil or grease after shaving. They should have following characteristics:

i) They should not be too thick or too thin.
ii) They should spread easily over the face in a thin film.

iii) They should be oily or lubricating during the shaving operations.
iv) They should make the beard soft.
v) They should be rinsed easily from the razor even with the cold water.
vi) They should be stable during their shelf life. There should not be any change, in their physical properties.
vii) They should possess a perfume to meet the masculine taste.

The usual materials to prepare brushless creams are stearic acid, caustic potash, glycerine, mineral oil, vegetable oil, wetting agents, boric acid, borax, triethanolamine and other amines, sulphonated oils, propylene glycols, alcohol, beeswax, spermaceti, cetyl alcohol, stearyl alcohol, lanolin etc. Apart from these materials, a suitable perfume is added to the formulation.

| Formula: Brushless Shaving Cream | |
|---|---|
| Stearic acid (XXX) | : 25 gm |
| Anhydrous lanolin | : 3 gm |
| Alcohol | : 2 ml |
| Triethanolamine | : 1 gm |
| Borax | : 0.5 gm |
| Glycerine | : 3 ml |
| Purified water | : 65 ml |
| Perfume | : ...q.s... |

Melt stearic acid and anhydrous lanolin in a water bath. Take triethanolamine, borax, glycerine and water in another beaker and heat upto 70°C. Add hot aqueous liquid to the melted portion with constant stirring. Stir until a smooth and white emulsion is formed. Add perfume dissolved in alcohol.

Lather shaving creams are semisolid preparations having proper consistency in order to exude from the collapsible tube easily without losing their physical form. They possess a unique property of producing abundant lather that does not dry on the face too rapidly, in addition to the characteristics of softening the beard and holding individual hair erect for close shaving. During shaving, lubricity for the razor is maintained thus making the shaving smooth and comfortable. They are economical for the user as less amount of cream per shave

# Cosmetics for Hair and Shaving Media

is required. They might have some other properties to improve their appeal like cooling sensation, antiseptic and astringent effects.

Materials like stearic acid, tallow, stearine, coconut oil, olive oil, peanut oil, caustic potash, caustic soda, glycerine, alcohol, lanolin, borax, boric acid, propylene glycol, aromatics etc., are employed to formulate a desired lather shaving cream.

| Formula: Lather Shaving Cream | |
|---|---|
| Stearic acid (XXX) | : 35.6 gm |
| Coconut oil | : 6.4 ml |
| Triethanolamine | : 1 gm |
| Glycerine | : 6 ml |
| Potassium hydroxide | : 7 gm |
| Sodium hydroxide | : 0.46 gm |
| Purified water | : 43 ml |
| Perfume | : …q.s… |

Melt stearic acid and add coconut oil in a beaker. Take water, glycerine, triethanolamine, potassium and sodium hydroxide in another beaker and heat on water bath to dissolve alkalis. Add melted stearic acid into hot alkali solution with constant stirring. Continue the stirring gently, not too rapidly, until a smooth cream is formed. When cool add perfume and mix.

# 4. COSMETICS FOR NAILS

**Cosmetics for Nails:**

Nails are protective covering of the fingers toes. They grow out of the cuticle or horny layer of the skin. Thus, it is necessary to take care of this growth which can create an odd situation if not been taken care of. The care of nails is referred to as manicuring.

Manicure preparations include many preparations like nail polish or enamel, polish remover, powder polish, paste polish, nail cream, nail bleach, cuticle remover, cuticle softener and nail tint. Out of these products, nails polishes have earned more popularity amongst the women as an important component of their make-up box.

Nail polishes consist of a base, like triacetyl cellulose or nitrocellulose, a resin, a plasticizer, a solvent, a dye and a suitable perfume.

Nitrocellulose, if added alone, forms a brittle film, would not spread properly on the nail. Thus, few resins and plasticizers are likely to be added. Solvents used, must have character that the lacquer should have been set in about a minute after application, acetone, alcohol, amyl acetate, ethyl acetate, amyl formate and ethyl propionate are used in combination or alone as solvents. Pigments must comply with the terms of the Food and Cosmetic Act. As such perfume is not necessary in nail enamels but some may add to make it specific product.

| Formula: Nail Enamel | |
|---|---|
| Nitrocellulose | : 10 gm |
| Ethyl acetate | : 55 gm |
| Butyl acetate | : 20 gm |
| Diethyl phthalate | : 10 gm |
| Camphor | : 4 gm |
| Colour | : ...q.s... |

Dissolve the nitrocellulose and the camphor in the ethyl acetate. Add the rest of the ingredients along with colour and perfume. Mix well.

# Cosmetics for Nails

Before application of nail enamel, finger nails must not possess even a slight impressions of old coatings of enamel in order to apply a fresh enamel smooth and uniformly spread. Thus, the nails must be rubbed with nail enamel remover with the help of cotton plug. Nail polish removers can be prepared with either single solvents like acetone or combination of solvents of which the following formula is popular.

| Formula: Nail Polish Remover | |
|---|---|
| Butyl stearate | : 60 gm |
| Ethyl stearate | : 40 gm |

Mix well the two ingredients.

## 5. DENTIFRICES

**Dentifrices:**

No doubt, dentifrices are being produced by some cosmetic manufacturers but in reality they are not cosmetic products. They are more or less related with the hygiene of the body parts, i.e. mouth cavity, thus can easily be put under hygienic products. They are necessary to cleanse the oral cavity including teeth. They also counteract bad breadth and leave a refreshing clean taste in the mouth. Cleaning of teeth is now-a-days becoming a part of a procedure for improving the personality and good health.

Dentifrices are available in the form of paste and powder. Their application is carried out with the help of tooth brush or the fingers of hand. An ideal dentifrices must have following qualities:

i) It must clean the teeth, remove the oily surface, or debris from the surface of the teeth.
ii) It must reduce the tooth decay.
iii) It must remove bad odour of the mouth cavity.
iv) It must improve the health of gums and makes them healthy.
v) It must provide good flavour in the mouth as an after effect.

There are number of ingredients required to make dentifrices possessing the above characteristics:

**1) Polishing agents (Abrasives):**

These agents possess the property of abrasiveness which helps them to act as polishing agents or as debris removers. Commonly precipitated calcium carbonate, tribasic calcium phosphate, calcium pyrophosphate, hydrated alumina, magnesium trisilicate etc. are used.

**2) Surface active agents (Detergents):**

They are known for their detergent action in order to enhance the action of polishing agents by wetting the teeth. Debris particles might be emulsified in the mouth cavity with the

# Dentifrices

help of surface active agent and can easily be removed from mouth cavity. They include sodium lauryl sulphate, sodium sulphosuccinate etc.

### 3) Humectants:

Humectants have the characteristic to keep the tooth-paste moist in order to protect it from drying which might create an odd condition while taking out the paste from the tube. Most commonly used humectants are glycerine, sorbitol, propylene glycol etc. Generally, 5 to 10% of humectants is preferred to add into a dentifrice paste.

### 4) Binders:

They are again important ingredients of a tooth paste where they are added to keep the solids and liquids united. They include gum tragacanth, gum karaya, sodium alginate, methyl cellulose etc. Usually 1 to 3% binders are added.

### 5) Sweetening agents:

They are added to impart a sweet taste to the dentifrices. Commonly used sweetening agent is saccharin in the concentration of 0.005 to 0.25%.

### 6) Flavouring agents:

These are the most important ingredients for dentifrices since most of the people always confirm the flavour of paste and powder before purchasing any of them. They are able to provide good flavour in the mouth cavity after its cleansing and maintaining it for a period of time. The most commonly used flavouring agents are peppermint oil, winter green oil, cinnamon oil etc. Usually, 0.5 to 2% flavouring agents can be added to the formula.

### 7) Preservatives:

Particularly in case of paste, preservatives are necessary to add into formulation in order to preserve the paste containing carbohydrates along with enough moisture content for bacterial growth. Commonly used preservatives are methyl and propyl paraben.

### 8) Miscellaneous agents:

Sometimes tooth pastes or powders are made medicated to provide some specific action. So some therapeutic agents are also added to the formulations to check the dental diseases. They may be bactericidal, bacteriostatic enzymes inhibiting agents or acids

# Dentifrices

neutralizing agents are used in medicated tooth pastes. Commonly used medicinal agents are fluorides, chlorophyll, urea, dibasic ammonium phosphate etc. Medicated tooth pastes must not be encouraged for daily use.

| Formula - I: Tooth Paste | |
|---|---|
| Precipitated chalk (light) | : 50 gm |
| Colloidal clay | : 4 gm |
| Tragacanth mucilage (2%) | : 3 gm |
| Glucose | : 2 gm |
| Glycerine | : 10 ml |
| Purified water | : 30.3 ml |
| Methyl paraben | : 0.2 gm |
| Peppermint oil | : 0.5 ml |

Dissolve glucose in water. To this add glycerine and tragacanth mucilage. Separately sift precipitated chalk and colloidal clay through fine sieve. Mix the two powders uniformly and then incorporate the powder mixture slowly with the liquid mixture with constant stirring until a smooth paste is obtained. Then add methyl paraben and peppermint oil. Mix them thoroughly.

| Formula - II: Tooth Paste (With Detergent) | |
|---|---|
| Dicalcium phosphate | : 35 gm |
| Calcium carbonate | : 19 gm |
| Glycerine | : 15 ml |
| Gum tragacanth | : 1.2 gm |
| Saccharine | : 0.05 gm |
| Sodium Lauryl Sulphate | : 18.25 gm |
| Flavour | : ...q.s... |

Mix glycerine with water. To this add solid ingredients which have been already passed through fine sieve, with constant stirring. Then add flavour. Mix thoroughly.

# Dentifrices

| **Formula - III: Tooth Powder** | |
|---|---|
| Precipitated calcium carbonate | : 75 gm |
| Hard soap, powdered | : 15 gm |
| Methyl salicylate | : 6 gm |
| Peppermint oil | : 2 ml |
| Cinnamon oil | : 1.5 ml |
| Saccharine | : ...q.s... |

Sift the solid ingredients through fine sieve and mix them in ascending order. Then add methyl salicylate, peppermint oil and cinnamon oil. Mix thoroughly to get uniform mixture. Again pass the mixture through fine sieve to remove the lumps, if any.

# Bibliography

**BIBLIOGRAPHY**

- *British National Formulary,* 51st edn (2006) London: BMJ Publishing Group and RPS Publishing.
- *British Pharmaceutical Codex* (1968) London: Pharmaceutical Press.
- *British Pharmaceutical Codex* (1973) London: Pharmaceutical Press.
- *British Pharmacopoeia* (1980) London: HMSO.
- *British Pharmacopoeia* (1988) London: HMSO.
- *British Pharmacopoeia* (2004) London: TSO.
- Marriott J F, Wilson K A, Langley C A, Belcher D (2006) *Pharmaceutical Compounding and Dispensing.* London: Pharmaceutical Press.
- *Martindale. The Extra Pharmacopoeia,* 26th edn. (1972) London: Pharmaceutical Press.
- *Martindale. The Extra Pharmacopoeia,* 31st edn. (1996) London: Royal Pharmaceutical Society.
- *Martindale. The Complete Drug Reference,* 33rd edn. (2002) London: Pharmaceutical Press.
- Aulton M E, ed (1988) *Pharmaceutics – The Science of Dosage for Design.* Edinburgh: Churchill Livingstone.
- Banker G S, Rhodes C T, ed (2002) *Modern Pharmaceutics.* New York: Marcel Dekker.
- Collett D M, Aulton M E, eds (1990) *Pharmaceutical Practice.* Edinburgh: Churchill Livingstone.
- Florence A T, Attwood D (1998) *Physicochemical Principles of Pharmacy.* Hampshire: Palgrave.
- Ghosh T K, Jasti B R, eds (2005) *Theory and Practice of Contemporary Pharmaceutics.* Florida: CRC Press.
- Rees J A, Smith I, Smith B (2001) *Introduction to Pharmaceutical Calculations.* London: Pharmaceutical Press.
- Anderson S, ed (2005) *Making Medicines: A Brief History of Pharmacy and Pharmaceuticals.* London: Pharmaceutical Press.

# More Books!

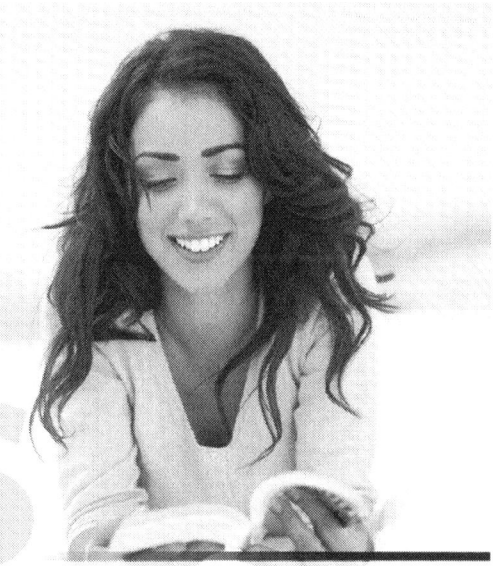

# I want morebooks!

Buy your books fast and straightforward online - at one of the world's fastest growing online book stores! Environmentally sound due to Print-on-Demand technologies.

Buy your books online at
**www.get-morebooks.com**

Kaufen Sie Ihre Bücher schnell und unkompliziert online – auf einer der am schnellsten wachsenden Buchhandelsplattformen weltweit! Dank Print-On-Demand umwelt- und ressourcenschonend produziert.

Bücher schneller online kaufen
**www.morebooks.de**

OmniScriptum Marketing DEU GmbH
Bahnhofstr. 28
D - 66111 Saarbrücken
Telefax: +49 681 93 81 567-9

info@omniscriptum.com
www.omniscriptum.com

Printed in Great Britain
by Amazon